RESPIRATORY SYNCTIAL VIRUS IN CHILDREN

UNDERSTANDING THE NATURE OF RESPIRATORY SYNCTIAL VIRUS IN CHILDREN

DR. J. WALLER

Contents

INTRODUCTION

A common viral infection that mostly affects the respiratory system, respiratory syncytial virus (RSV) is more frequent in newborns and young children. An overview of RSV in children is given here:

A common cause of respiratory tract infections, particularly in young children, is the Paramyxoviridae family virus known as respiratory Syncytial virus (RSV). All ages are susceptible to RSV infections, but small children especially those under the age of two are most vulnerable.

Important Points:

Transfer:

When an infected person coughs or sneezes, respiratory droplets are released into the air, making RSV extremely contagious. Additionally, it can be acquired by coming into contact with infected surfaces.

Time of Year:

Seasonal epidemics of RSV infections are common, usually occurring in the fall and winter. Widespread outbreaks of the virus can occur in homes, schools, and childcare facilities.

Signs:

Children's RSV symptoms can vary from minor cold-like symptoms like fever, runny nose, and cough to more serious respiratory conditions including pneumonia and bronchiolitis. In severe cases, breathing difficulties and wheezing are prevalent.

High-Risk Entities:

Severe problems from RSV are more likely among prematurely born infants, people with congenital heart disease, people with long-term lung diseases, and those with compromised immune systems.

Avoidance:

Since there is no particular antiviral therapy for RSV, prophylaxis is essential. Avoiding direct contact with sick people, washing your hands frequently, and maintaining clean shared surfaces are among preventative measures.

Bedding in:

Hospitalization may be necessary for severe RSV infections, particularly in young children. Children in hospitals may require supportive treatment, such as intravenous fluids and oxygen therapy.

Immunity Development:

Serious infections are more prevalent in the first few years of birth, even though RSV reinfections are common throughout life. As people age, their immunity tends to increase, offering some defense against serious illness from following illnesses.

Recognizing the common symptoms, risk factors, and preventive strategies is essential to understanding RSV in children. Early intervention and medical care are critical, especially in high-risk populations, as is the case with any respiratory infection. Research on RSV is also ongoing, with the goal of developing effective treatment and prevention plans for this prevalent children sickness.

CHAPTER ONE

Spread and Transmission in Children

Children contract the respiratory syncytial virus (RSV) mostly from direct contact with respiratory droplets. An outline of how RSV spreads among kids is provided below:

Breathing Droplets:

RSV is most often spread by respiratory droplets that are released when an infected person talks, sneezes, or coughs. People in the vicinity may inhale these droplets, which may contain the virus.

Direct Communication:

Direct contact with an infected person's respiratory secretions can potentially spread RSV. This can occur when kids share personal objects like toys or touch their face after coming into contact with infected surfaces.

Polluted Surfaces:

RSV can last for several hours on surfaces. Children can get infected by touching their face, particularly their mouth, nose, or eyes, after coming into contact with a surface or object that has the RSV virus on it.

Communal Environments:

Due to close contact and shared areas, places where children congregate like playgrounds, schools, and daycare centers are favorable to the spread of RSV.

Periodic Epidemics:

Seasonal epidemics of RSV infections are common, usually occurring in the fall and winter. In cooler climates, the virus spreads more readily.

Transmission in the Home:

RSV is frequently spread among family members in homes, particularly between siblings. The virus is more likely to propagate in close quarters.

Extremely Contagious Character

It is difficult to stop the spread of RSV in public places since the virus is extremely contagious and affected youngsters can shed it for a long time.

Keeping children clean and taking preventative action are key to preventing the spread of RSV in children:

Handwashing Frequently: Teach kids to wash their hands with soap and water on a regular basis, especially after handling objects or coughing or sneezing.

Children should be taught to cover their mouth and nose when coughing or sneezing by using a tissue or their elbow, according to respiratory etiquette.

Minimize Close Contact: Keep healthy and sick youngsters away from one other. This is especially crucial in environments that include childcare.

Cleaning and disinfecting: To lower the danger of surface transfer, clean and disinfect shared products, toys, and surfaces that are commonly touched on a regular basis.

Parents, caregivers, and daycare providers can lessen the risk of RSV transmission in children by putting these precautions into practice.

Children's Symptoms and Signs

Children infected with the respiratory syncytial virus (RSV) may experience mild cold-like symptoms or more severe respiratory distress. The following are typical indications and symptoms of RSV in kids:

Cough

One of the primary signs of RSV in children is a chronic cough. It could begin as a moderate cough and get worse over time.

Runny nose:

Like the ordinary cold, nasal congestion and runny nose are frequent early symptoms of RSV.

Temperature spike:

When they have RSV, many kids get feverish. The fever might range in intensity from low to severe.

Sneezing:

Sneezing is a common symptom of RSV infection in children and helps transmit the virus.

Sighing:

Children with RSV frequently wheeze, a high-pitched whistling sound made when breathing, particularly when bronchiolitis is present.

Inability to Breathe:

In more serious situations, kids could have trouble breathing or breathe quickly. It occurs more frequently in babies.

Breathiness Shortness:

Breathlessness can be brought on by RSV, especially in younger children and those with underlying respiratory disorders.

Bluish skin, or cyanosis:

In extreme circumstances, oxygen deprivation can cause cyanosis, a blue color to the lips and skin.

Intolerance:

Due to respiratory pain, children with RSV may become irritable and have difficulty falling asleep.

Diminished Hunger:

Children who are impacted by respiratory symptoms and discomfort may experience a decrease in appetite.

It's crucial to remember that RSV symptoms can mimic those of other respiratory illnesses, making it difficult to distinguish between them just by looking at symptoms. RSV can result in bronchiolitis in newborns, which is an inflammation of the lungs' tiny airways and can cause more serious symptoms.

When a kid exhibits respiratory distress, frequent coughing, or other indications of dehydration, parents and other caregivers should take them to the doctor. Medical attention and early management can help control the symptoms and lower the chance of consequences.

A combination of clinical examination, medical history, and, in certain situations, laboratory testing is usually used in the diagnosis and assessment of Respiratory Syncytial Virus (RSV) in children. The following is how medical practitioners can go about diagnosing and assessing RSV in children:

Clinical Evaluation:

Medical History: The doctor will ask about the child's symptoms, including fever, coughing, and any indications of respiratory distress. They will also ask about the beginning and course of the child's respiratory symptoms.

Physical Examination: To evaluate the child's respiratory symptoms, a comprehensive physical examination is carried out, which includes listening to the lungs for wheezing or crackles.

Laboratory Examinations:

Nasal or Throat Swab: To check for the presence of RSV, a swab sample from the nose or throat may be taken. Polymerase chain reaction (PCR) testing or rapid antigen tests are frequently used to identify the virus.

Nasopharyngeal Aspirate: A small, flexible tube called a "nasopharyngeal aspirate" may be used in some situations to gather a sample of mucus from the back of the nose and throat for laboratory testing.

Blood Examinations:

Although less common than swab tests, blood tests may be performed in specific circumstances to assess for the presence of RSV antibodies.

Chest X-ray:

An X-ray of the chest may be used to determine the extent of lung involvement if the kid has severe respiratory symptoms or pneumonia-like indications.

Oximetry of the pulse:

A pulse oximeter can be used to measure oxygen saturation, particularly when respiratory distress is a potential issue.

Assessment of Intensity:

Based on the child's age, underlying medical conditions, and symptoms, healthcare professionals determine the severity of RSV infection.

RSV diagnosis in children is frequently made using a combination of laboratory test results and clinical presentation. Quick results from rapid diagnostic testing can help with prompt action and suitable care.

It's critical that parents or other adult caregivers get a kid medical help if they show signs of respiratory distress, such as wheezing, cyanosis, or rapid breathing. Early diagnosis lowers the risk of consequences from severe RSV infections and enables the provision of appropriate supportive care, particularly in newborns.

In order to lower the chance of transmission, hygienic practices and protective measures are combined to prevent children from contracting Respiratory Syncytial Virus (RSV). The following are important methods for preventing RSV in children:

Hand Sanitization:

Encourage people to wash their hands often with soap and water, especially after touching surfaces, sneezing, or coughing. If soap and water are not available, use hand sanitizers with alcohol base.

CHAPTER TWO

Pneumonia Etiquette:

When your child coughs or sneezes, teach them to cover their mouth and nose with a tissue or their elbow. Discourage them from covering their mouths with their hands.

Steer clear of close contact:

Restrict the amount of time that sick and well children spend together, particularly in public places like childcare facilities and schools.

Empty and Rinse:

Clean and sanitize shared products, toys, and surfaces that are regularly touched on a regular basis. RSV can last for several hours on surfaces.

Steer clear of shared items:

Prohibit sharing of personal objects such as toys, glasses, and cutlery, particularly in places where kids hang out.

Immunization (if accessible):

RSV has no readily accessible vaccination as of January 2022, when I last updated my understanding. Still, current studies are investigating the creation of vaccines for elderly people as well as newborns.

Reducing Exposure:

Reduce the amount of time you spend with those who have respiratory infections. Avoid crowded areas when RSV is prevalent, especially with young children.

Nursing:

Encourage breastfeeding if at all possible. Antibodies from breast milk can aid in preventing respiratory infections in babies.

Optimal Respiratory Care:

Teach kids the importance of respiratory hygiene, including how to properly dispose of tissues and use tissues to wipe their noses.

Seasonal Sensitivity:

Recognize that RSV outbreaks follow seasonal patterns, usually occurring in the fall and winter. Aim for extra safety during these times.

In order to put these preventive measures into practice, parents and other caregivers are essential. When RSV is more common, it's crucial to be on the lookout for respiratory symptoms in children and to get them medical help, especially if they are having trouble breathing or showing indications of dehydration.

Methods of Therapy for Children

Since there is no specific antiviral medicine approved for treating RSV infections in children, the primary treatment for RSV in children is supportive care. The following are typical methods for treating RSV in children:

Symptomatic Management:

Acetaminophen or ibuprofen are examples of over-the-counter drugs that can be used to treat fever and discomfort. Use these drugs, therefore, only under a doctor's supervision.

Nasal Aspiration:

Nasal suctioning can help babies breathe easier and eliminate mucus, especially if they have congestion in their noses.

Drinking plenty of water

Make sure the child is getting enough fluids, especially if they are susceptible to dehydration from a fever, poor appetite, or respiratory distress.

Relax:

Give the kid enough sleep so that they can heal more quickly. Better sleep and general wellbeing can be enhanced by a calm and cozy setting.

Air that has been humidified:

Add moisture to the air in the child's room with a humidifier to assist ease coughing and congestion in the nose.

Keeping an eye on the respiratory state:

Keep an eye on the child's breathing effort and rate. If you have symptoms of respiratory distress, such as rapid breathing, wheezing, or difficulty breathing, get medical help.

Treatment using Oxygen:

Extra oxygen therapy may be given in a hospital setting in extreme cases where respiratory distress is substantial.

Inpatient care (if necessary):

Severe RSV infections may necessitate hospitalization for intensive observation and supportive care, particularly in newborns and kids with underlying medical issues.

It's crucial to remember that viruses like RSV cannot be treated with drugs. The goal of treatment is to help the kid heal by controlling symptoms and offering supportive care.

To lower the risk of RSV transmission in children, preventive steps like practicing good hand hygiene, avoiding direct contact with sick people, and keeping a clean environment are essential.

In the event that a child exhibits symptoms of a serious illness, respiratory distress, or serious dehydration, parents and caregivers should seek immediate medical help. Medical experts can offer advice on proper treatment and observation during the disease.

Pediatric Populations at High Risk

It is thought that some child populations are more vulnerable to serious consequences from respiratory syncytial virus (RSV) infections. Among these at-risk demographics are:

Young Children and Infants:

Severe RSV infections are more common in children under the age of one, especially in preterm babies. Infants born too soon may not have fully developed respiratory and immune systems.

Youngsters with Prolonged Lung Diseases:

Children who have long-term respiratory problems like bronchopulmonary dysplasia (BPD) or asthma are at a higher risk of developing severe RSV infections.

Congenital heart disease in children:

If infected with RSV, those who have congenital heart disease may face more severe symptoms and problems.

Youngsters with Immune System Impairments:

Severe RSV infections are more common in kids with compromised immune systems, whether as a result of illnesses like HIV/AIDS or immunosuppressive drugs like those used after transplants.

Youngsters Affected by Neuromuscular Disorders:

Children who suffer from diseases that affect respiratory muscle function, such as muscular dystrophy or other neuromuscular problems, are more vulnerable to respiratory infections, such as RSV.

Kids in Congested Environments:

People who live in crowded environments, including childcare facilities or homes with several siblings, may be more susceptible to contracting RSV.

Offspring of Smoking Mothers:

Pregnant women who smoke may put their unborn children at greater risk of developing serious RSV infections.

Specific ethnic groupings

The causes of certain research' findings that specific ethnic groups might be more susceptible to severe RSV infections remain unclear.

To protect high-risk pediatric groups from RSV, preventive steps are essential. These include practicing good hand hygiene, avoiding close contact with sick people, and receiving vaccinations when available. Furthermore, RSV prophylaxis may be advised by medical professionals, particularly for preterm babies or patients with certain illnesses that make them more susceptible to severe RSV disease.

Children's Complications and Long-Term Impacts

Although severe infections might result in difficulties, the majority of instances of Respiratory Syncytial Virus (RSV) in children are mild and self-limiting. The following are possible long-term consequences and difficulties linked to RSV in children:

CHAPTER THREE

Bronchiolitis:

Bronchiolitis, or inflammation of the tiny airways in the lungs, is frequently caused by RSV. Breathing difficulties, wheezing, and coughing may follow from this.

Pneumonia:

Severe RSV infections have the potential to develop into lung infections called pneumonia. Breathing difficulties, a high fever, and chest pain are all possible signs of pneumonia.

After contracting RSV, children with a history of asthma may see an increase in their symptoms.

Infections of the ears:

Otitis media, or middle ear infections, can result from RSV infections, particularly in younger children.

Breathing Pauses, or Apnea:

RSV-infected babies, especially those who are born prematurely, may have apnea, a condition in which infants briefly stop breathing.

Bedding in:

Severe RSV infections may necessitate hospitalization for intensive observation and supportive care, particularly in infants and children at high risk.

Breathing Problems:

Respiratory distress in children might manifest as wheezing, fast breathing, and increased strain of breathing.

Dehydration:

Dehydration may be a concern for children with RSV, particularly if they are vomiting frequently or are not drinking as much fluids.

Effects of Long-Term Respiratory:

While the majority of kids recover completely from RSV, some could have respiratory symptoms like coughing and wheezing that last for weeks or even months.

Enhanced Vulnerability to Additional Infections

Children who have RSV infections are more vulnerable to other respiratory illnesses because they have a weakened immune system.

It's crucial to remember that high-risk groups, such as newborns, kids with underlying medical issues, and premature babies, are more likely to experience serious consequences.

Reducing the risk of problems related to RSV requires early symptom assessment, preventive interventions, and rapid medical attention. If a kid exhibits indications of respiratory distress or if the condition is severe, parents and other caretakers should take them to the doctor. Depending on the severity of the condition, medical specialists can offer the right advice and treatment.

Coping Mechanisms for Parents and Guardians

It can be difficult for parents and other caregivers to deal with children who have respiratory syncytial virus (RSV). Here are some coping mechanisms to aid in getting through the situation:

Remain Up to Date:

Find out more about RSV, its symptoms, and how long the infection should last. Being aware of what to anticipate might reduce anxiety.

Interact with Healthcare Professionals:

Keep lines of communication open with medical professionals. Talk to your child's doctor about any worries you may have regarding their symptoms and course of treatment.

Establish a Cozy Environment

Make sure your child is at ease by setting up a calm environment. To relieve congestion, use a humidifier and surround yourself with cozy things like a plush blanket or toy.

Promote Hydration

Offer your youngster fluids on a regular basis to help them keep hydrated. Preventing dehydration is crucial, particularly in cases where your child has a fever.

Keep an eye on your symptoms:

Pay special attention to your child's symptoms and get help if you encounter any indications of respiratory distress, a prolonged fever, or other worrisome symptoms.

Sleep and Rest:

Make sure your child gets enough sleep so that their body can heal. A child who gets enough sleep is better able to fight off the virus.

Offer Emotional Assistance:

Provide your youngster with comfort and emotional support. Tell them you're here to support them when they're sick.

Depend on Your Support Network:

Seek emotional assistance from friends, family, or support organizations. It might be consoling to share experiences with those who have gone through comparable circumstances.

Observe Self-Care:

Never forget to look after your own health. To keep mentally and physically strong, make sure you manage stress, eat a balanced diet, and get adequate sleep.

Observe Medical Advice

Observe the advice of medical specialists and adhere to the treatment plan. If you are provided medication, take it as instructed.

Remain Upbeat:

Pay attention to the good parts of your child's healing and improvement. Honor little successes and accomplishments.

It's important to keep in mind that different people have different coping mechanisms, so you and your child should figure out what works best for you both. Do not hesitate to seek out additional support from mental health or medical specialists if you are feeling overwhelmed. They can offer counsel specific to your circumstance.

CONCLUSION

In conclusion, respiratory symptoms ranging from moderate to severe are caused by the common viral infection known as Respiratory Syncytial Virus (RSV), which primarily affects newborns and young children. While severe infections can result in consequences, particularly in high-risk populations, the majority of RSV cases in children resolve on their own.

A clean environment, avoiding direct contact with sick people, practicing excellent hand hygiene, and other preventive actions are essential in lowering the risk of RSV transmission in children. When available, vaccination programs seek to offer further defense against serious RSV infections.

Managing RSV in children requires parents and caregivers to be knowledgeable about the condition, recognize symptoms early, and seek medical help promptly when needed. A soothing atmosphere, hydration, and symptom treatment are examples of supportive care that helps a kid heal.

When RSV infections occur, high-risk groups such as newborns, people with underlying medical issues, and prematurely born babies need extra care and observation. Complication risk can be reduced by prompt action and following medical advice.

The creation of efficacious vaccinations and treatment interventions continues to be a priority in the endeavor to further enhance the

management and prevention of RSV in children
as long as research and medical developments
persist.

THE END